Listen To Your Body

By

Zanna Lee Sturm

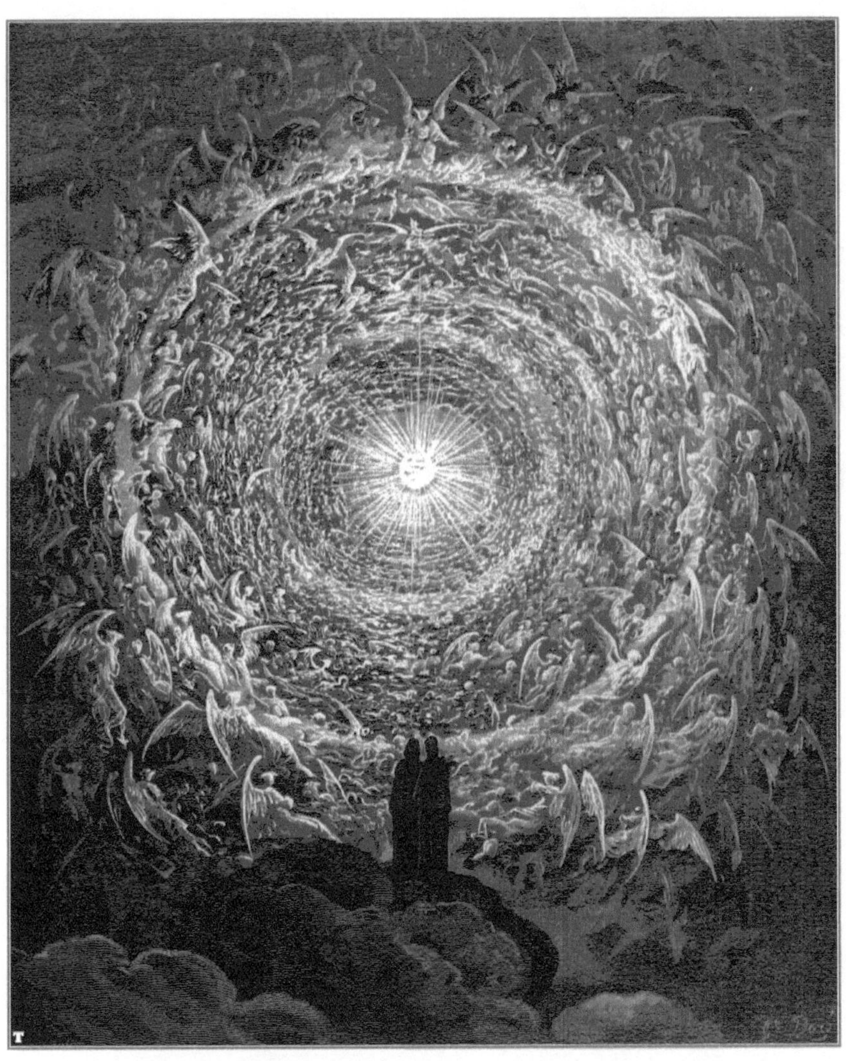

This book is inspired by my son Gabriel
whose strength is beyond measure,
whose will is beyond strength
and whose spirit will live on
forever.

TABLE OF CONTENTS

<u>**FORWARD**</u>

I am a firm believer that experience is our best teacher. The following healing regimen I am about to share with you stems from a 20-year journey of research, experience and experimentation with alternative and natural healing that hit the glass ceiling when my son was diagnosed with Crohn's Disease. The good news is, we broke that ceiling!

I have studied and practiced under many good teachers who made popular the holistic natural health and healing movement back in the 60's. From the raw food evangelists of Anne Wigmore and Viktorus Kulvinskis, to the soy fields of The Farm, I have tried many alternative diets and methods of cleansing including being a vegetarian for nearly 20 years, a devout raw foodist for 3 years and even being a fruitarian for 6 months after a rigorous 20 day fast. I have many knowledgeable friends and mentors of whom I have learned much from by asking questions, reading and researching a myriad of books and publications but mostly experimenting on myself.

Throughout my life, I have had lots of success in curing just about any ailment through nutritional therapy and cleansing. The sheer bravery of pushing further into curing Crohn's was based solely on the successes I have had with my own history in healing, intuition and a strong will as this time it was not my own body I was trying to heal, but my sons.

I am in no way a doctor although I do consider myself a healer. I in no way guarantee that these methods will heal you of your disease although I can claim that if these recommendations are followed diligently, you will experience a healthier more pleasant existence and an improved state of being.

It is also essential that you stick with the diet, supplementation and suggested therapies for at least 6 months or until you are fully healed for maximum results. It took us 2 years.

What works for one person may not work for another. We are all unique with different lifestyles, blood types and DNA. But fundamentally, we all come from a common source. The closer we live with the Earth and the natural World, the closer we will be to perfect health.

Most of all, listen to your body! It talks to you on a daily basis. Things that are good for you feel good. Things that are not good create unsavory conditions in the body such as cramps, anxiety, headaches, tiredness or anything contradictory to a state of well-being. If you listen to your body, it will guide you in what you need to heal and live a healthy life.

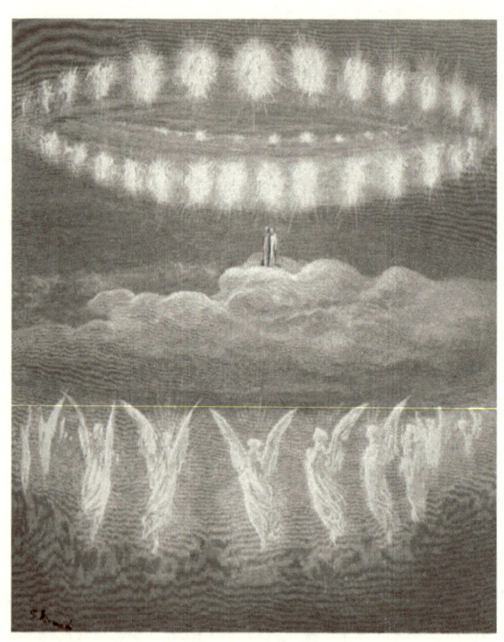

<u>**OUR STORY**</u>

Our story began long ago when I discovered herbal medicine. I was reading a book series that documented how our ancestors used plants to heal all manner of ailments. I was fascinated and took a trip to the health food store where I immediately landed a job in the herb department. The rest is history. For over 30 years now, I have dabbled with herbs, nutritional therapy and alternative remedies where I have discovered that many ailments can be cured from the comfort of your own kitchen or local health food store. I have studied many alternative diets that emphasize only eating whole, unprocessed foods from the Earth. I have tried many flavors of vegetarianism including: macrobiotic, vegan, raw food and fruitarian. I learned a lot from these diets but it was my 3 year stint of being a devout raw foodist that taught me the most about how food is the real medicine as it incorporates regular cleansing and fasting along with living foods. I could cure just about any ailment using plants, cleansing methods and raw food. I prided myself in not having to go to a doctor when I had a common ailment.

Then my son got very sick. We had gone rafting on the Nantahala River and had brought some snacks for the ride. While I was handing my son some yogurt, the raft guide insisted he stick it in the river to get it cold. That ended up being the worst mistake of our lives. I later found out that the Nantahala is one of the most polluted rivers in the country.   He threw up the entire way home and didn't stop for what seemed like months. At first I thought it was food poisoning and tried everything I knew to heal him but after days of no success, I knew he needed a doctor. After multiple trips and several weeks of both alternative and allopathic medicine, his condition only worsened. He had dropped 30 pounds in 3 months, wouldn't eat and kept losing weight. The doctor could not figure out what was wrong with him. She finally referred us to a specialist who immediately diagnosed him with Crohn's Disease; a debilitating, non-curable (or so they say) condition of the intestines where it is extremely painful to eat or absorb nutrients because the intestine is riddled with large sores that resemble holes. I know this because my son's doctor had him swallow a small camera to see the condition of his intestines and it looked like Billy the Kid had unleashed his rifle in there.

I believed that this condition was way out of my league as a healer and for the sake of my son's life and health decided to go the traditional

route. We had some mild success with drugs but when the doctor suggested chemo therapy and/or surgery for my son's worsening condition, I begged him to give me more time to keep trying some alternative means to heal my son. I had been researching and trying different things this whole time and had just reconnected with some of my old raw food friends who had some great advice about using a diet rich in probiotics. He agreed to give me two months to try these other methods before moving to a more extreme treatment such as surgery.
I immediately took my son off of all dairy, gluten and sugar including fruit and honey. I introduced an entirely new diet regimen rich in probiotics and nurturing bone broth and continued with an onslaught of herbal medicine consisting of natural antibiotics and plant based anti-inflammatory supplements. I also introduced colon cleansing through hydro-therapy with colonics and enemas.

Sure enough, after several weeks with this new diet and protocol, my son's doctor said "Whatever you are doing, keep doing it because his inflammation is down and he is getting better!"

Then, low and behold, I lost my insurance. This ended up being the best thing that ever happened to us.

Two years and loads of alternative therapies later, my son was completely cured of Crohn's Disease and has been symptom free for nearly 10 years.

This is our story.

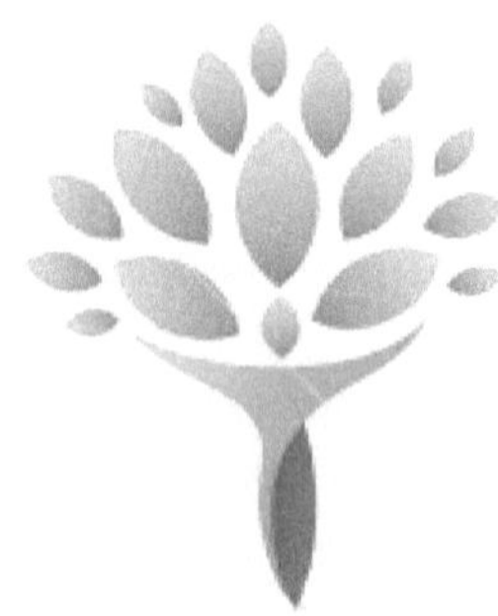

<u>**INTRODUCTION**</u>

I have to tell you that there will be doctors who will say there is no cure for Crohn's Disease. They will argue with you about most of what you will read in this book. These same doctors told me there was no cure and that my son would have to live with this disease for the rest of his life. Well, they were wrong! Although doctor's have their place, there is no one on this planet that knows your body better than you do. If you trust your intuition and really check the signs your body is giving you, you can find a method that works. I am mostly referring to diet, supplementation, therapies and all of the alternative means available.
Of course, this book is not intended to replace your doctor and you need to be conscious of where you are at with your disease because there are varying states of it and in severe cases, you need to stay on your prescribed medication until you reach a certain level of healing. It is all about balance. I suggest you do both traditional and alternative methods until you know you are in a good place to transition over.

Here is my hypothesis about Crohn's Disease based on my experience with my son. I believe that it is a super bacteria that scientists do not know how to kill. Think about it. There are new species of animals found every year both in the ocean and on land. With over 70 billion varieties, bacteria make up the largest population of species on the planet. There is no way humanly possible that we can know everything that exists on this Earth as things are always evolving, changing and living in some environments we cannot access.

The Nantahala River is laden with pesticides, fertilizers, chlorine, laundry soap and a myriad of other chemicals that wash off into the river every time it rains. Species evolve according to their environment. Who's to say that some bacteria haven't evolved to withstand this type of onslaught coming into their environment?   Even scientists have predicted a "Super Flu" brewing due to the overuse of antibiotics and bacteria becoming resistant to it.

I have absolutely no proof on my hypothesis other than logic and experience. Ironically, an article came out last year from a scholarly journal stating "Scientists Believe Crohn's is Caused by a Bacteria". I was thrilled when I saw this because my intuition had been telling me this from the beginning!   I deduced my bacteria hypothesis because I ultimately eradicated this disease using natural antibiotics. This however was not as simple as it may seem. This is a "super" bacteria. It took two long years of rigorous diet, therapy and supplementation to get rid of it! That's because the intestines are so injured from the disease and the friendly bacteria is so debilitated, they are vulnerable to further infection and it is very difficult to turn around the onslaught of bad bacteria attacking and making the situation worse.

There are two main things one must do to heal from this disease. Heal the intestines and kill the bacteria. This is not easy as in severe cases like my son the intestines can be pretty beaten up making them susceptible to further infection and sensitive to many things. It is a slow process but over time and with the right focus, it can be done.

The following chapters outline everything we did over this two year period. Keep in mind that we continued using the pharmaceutical drugs prescribed for the first few months before completely switching to alternative therapy and slowly weaned him off of them as his intestines began to heal.

Only you know when this time is right so as I have said and will say again, Listen to Your Body!

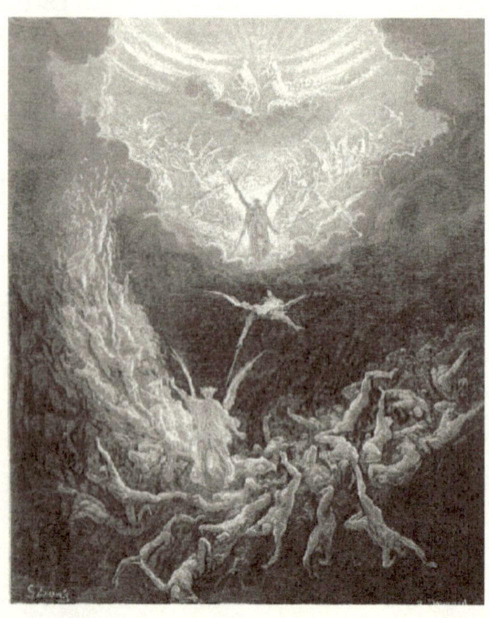

THE PHILOSOPHY

Water is the staff of life. This statement could not be more true as our bodies are made up mostly of water. The average amount of water that makes up a body is 57 percent of our total body weight although it can vary between 50-65 percent depending on your lifestyle and environment. In a newborn infant, this may be as high as 79 percent, but it progressively decreases from birth to old age.

This is an important fact because water in today's modern society has been severely compromised. Regular tap water is loaded with heavy chlorine, chemicals and debris that wipe out the friendly bacteria in our body and debilitate the body's natural method of detoxification. This combination alone compromises our immune system and creates a perfect environment for all kinds of disease. In fact, chemically laden water which is intended to cleanse our tissue only adds to the toxins already present within our bodies that come from air pollution, pesticides and chemicals present in all kinds of products and food we consume daily. On top of that, our filtered water is devoid of minerals that used to be present when our ancestors bathed in lakes and streams and drank from local springs. Magnesium is one of the key ingredients our bodies need to detox and many people in todays society are deficient because we no longer live as they did.

Well what about bottled mineral water? Bottled water is put in plastic which gives off toxic fumes and poisons the "purified water" so many stores are selling. Often times this bottled "spring" water is coming from the same tap you use in your home!

I knew that water was a factor intuitively when my son got sick. Thinking it might be my pipes, I had a guy come out and test the water in my house. I was horrified at what he showed me as to the levels of chemicals and debris that even a small filter couldn't handle. I immediately put a large filter on the main water supply to our house so that even our showers were filtered from these harmful substances. Think about how much water we absorb through our skin. I had already stopped swimming in chlorinated pools years ago because of their huge levels of toxicity but now I was determined to eliminate as many toxins in the environment as possible.

Obviously, home filters are expensive but there are many out there that you can hook up to your sink that can be helpful and are far superior to buying bottled water. If bottled water is the only option, hard plastic is much safer than softer plastic as it does not release as much toxic gas. Also, avoid letting your plastic bottle lay in sunlight as the heat exacerbates the release of toxic gas into the water. You can taste it!

Distilled water is also a good option as that process eliminates a lot of toxins and debris and has an electro-magnetic effect to it. It should be noted however that distilling water leaches out important minerals from the body as well. This water is good periodically for pulling out toxins and infection.

Whatever method you use, just drink good, purified water to start and lots of it! Twice your body weight in ounces per day is a good protocol. I carry around a huge 1 gallon jug with me and chug it all day long. You can never drink too much water!

As for the minerals missing in your water, the most important one is magnesium. I'm not talking about the form that comes in a pill. The best form of magnesium supplementation is Magnesium Citrate. It comes in a powder form that is highly absorbable and quick acting.

Our cells in their resting state contain magnesium. When under stress, calcium enters into the nerve cells and makes muscles tense. When the stress has passed, magnesium pushes the calcium back out of the cells and everything relaxes. However, when there's not enough magnesium, calcium remains in the cells, prolonging stress and creating magnesium-deficiency symptoms such as fatigue, low energy; inability to sleep; muscle tension, spasms and cramps; anxiousness and nervousness; headaches; inflammation; constipation and abnormal heart rhythms.

For a person with Crohn's many of these symptoms are present. Magnesium citrate will help alleviate many of the symptoms of Crohn's and help the body naturally detox during the healing process. This is also good for anyone really!

Just mix 1 tablespoon of powder into cold water and drink 1 to 3 times a day.

THE DIET

Hippocrates once said "Let food be your medicine". When we eat whole, unprocessed, organic food from the Earth, it should have every vitamin, mineral and nutrient in it to sustain and maintain a healthy body. Unfortunately, much of our soil is depleted so we still need vitamin and mineral supplements to compensate for this. Organic produce tends to be grown in environments where composting and soil rejuvenation are practiced. It is not a bad idea to research the farms however and find local organic produce as it has the nutrients most suited for your environment.

Let's start with foods to avoid. These include anything that is low fat or "fat free" as it is some of the worst stuff you can put in your body. The fat in food actually helps to digest and assimilate the nutrients. Fat free products such as margarine contain trans-fat and often have the same components that are used in plastic, making it almost impossible to metabolize. This leads to clogging of the arteries and all sorts of health problems. Artificial sweetener is also horrible as it is laden with chemicals and has been linked to cardiac arrest as well as a myriad of other debilitating ailments. Aspartame is said to turn into formaldehyde inside of your stomach! Bottom line if it is not directly from the Earth, do not eat it!

Another thing to consider is how to cook your food. Too many people overcook especially vegetables and kill all the nutrients in it. It is best to eat your vegetables raw but if you must cook, lightly steamed or warmed is fine. I like to add my onions and garlic at the end so that they are warm but still raw. That way they retain their medicinal value of being a natural antibiotic and anti-parasitic. Meat on the other hand, especially chicken, should be fully cooked as harmful bacteria can be present.

If you must use a microwave, never, ever cook anything in there in plastic! Just like water in the sun, the plastic gives off harmful gases that saturate your food and have been linked to many kinds of cancer. If you must use one, cook in ceramic or glass only. Of course, the best way to cook or heat your food is on the stove as a microwave tends to kill a lot of the beneficial life energy in food.

Processed, pesticide laden food has much of the nutritional value stripped from it including the valuable enzymes needed to break down the food and use it for healthy digestion and energy. Much of our tired, obese population suffers because there is no nutritional value in this type of food. With little nutritional value, it creates a sensation of always being hungry which creates the 'grazing' habit of eating all day. What's worse is without live enzymes in processed food, there is nothing to help digest it. It stays in our colon, clogs us up and creates a toxic cesspool for all sorts of disease to crop up. The pesticides only add to the toxicity inside. This is why colon cancer is the leading cause of death in the United States. Keeping your colon clean and clear is essential for optimum health, especially with Crohn's Disease.

Most food off the shelf is also heavily laden with sugar which creates an acidic environment inside of the body and is a breeding ground for parasites and bad bacteria. Canned food introduces harmful metals like aluminum which is the leading cause of alzheimers disease. Canned food with acidic contents such as pineapple or tomatoes are the worst as the acid eats at the metal and mixes it in with the food even more so.

The key to healthy living and a healthy colon is to eat plenty of fresh, live, organic fruits and vegetables. There are many diets out there and lord knows I've tried many. Overall, I have found it is good to eat according to your blood type and go about 80% raw. I have type "O" which means the only source of iron my body can metabolize is red meat. After nearly 20 years of being a staunch vegetarian I decided to try it and low and behold, I felt much better. Only you know truly what is right for you.

So what if you have Crohn's Disease? This is particularly important as it attacks the intestines directly. The doctor will tell you to eliminate all fiber from your diet including raw vegetables only fiber is essential in cleaning out the colon. Bottom line: Listen to your body! It will tell you what you can and can't eat. Start out with gentle foods and build up over time to more fiber as your gut heals. The best food to start with is by making your own bone broth. You can use chicken, cow or fish bones for this. By simmering the bones on low for 8 to 12 hours, the marrow is extracted from the bones and is very nourishing to the nervous system and stomach. The nutrients are easily digested from the broth itself which can also be used to cook lots of different recipes such as soups, stews, rice and sauces. Start out with just the broth and add in any vegetables such as onions, garlic, carrots, zuchinni and squash to make a really nice soup. I like to add in meat toward the end for extra protein.

THE ELIMINATION DIET

Changing your diet after years of building up habits can be daunting. It is best to do it in steps and slowly wean yourself. The first thing you should eliminate is all processed sugar products and white flour. Refined sugar irritates the intestinal walls and feeds the bacteria. If you must have sweetener, honey or stevia are good natural substitutes. Also eating dried fruit is a good alternative to ice cream.

I recommend eliminating white flour products altogether as they tend to clog up the colon and can be difficult to digest. Although white bread may seem soft, it turns into glue inside your stomach. Sour Dough bread made from a real sour dough starter, however is sufficient as it has live enzymes in it that help break down the flour. As your stomach heals, you can try sprouted bread found in the freezer of the health food section. The sprouted wheat has enzymes that make it easier to digest. Rice flour is also good as it is much easier to digest and quite tasty. You can find a lot of these kinds of breads in the gluten-free section of the store.

I truthfully am not a huge advocate of the gluten-free craze. It may work for some people but most of the products are very brittle to eat and don't taste that great. I believe that it's not gluten people are allergic to but the pesticides in the wheat. Again, this is my intuition speaking so don't quote me on that and please go gluten-free if you wish. I just feel like a lot of those boxed health food products are just as processed as the junk food products and clog up your colon just as much only without the pesticides. If you must, read the label! Be conscious of what kind of flour and how much sugar is present. Live food from the Earth is always best.

Avoid heavy foods such as pasta and bread or any processed, boxed food you find on the shelf. As mentioned before, these are hard to digest as there aren't live enzymes in there to help. If you must eat these, take enzymes in pill form to compensate or eat some raw food with it. Rice flour products are best in my opinion if you need some carbs.

Do not eat vegetables that may be too rough to digest. These include hard veggies such as raw cabbage, kale and carrots. Although I am an advocate of raw, uncooked vegetables, if you suffer lots of pain when you eat, lightly steamed vegetables are good until you have healed up inside enough to handle the raw veggies. Raw spinach however can usually be tolerated.

The best method for eating vegetables when you have Crohn's is to juice them. Juicing your vegetables and fruits is an amazing way to get the nutrients without irritating the damaged areas of your intestines. Carrot-Beet juice is very cleansing for the blood and re-building of the tissue walls as are many other combinations. You can add raw ginger, tumeric and garlic to these to get even more benefits out of them as these are both anti-bacterial, anti-inflammatory and digestive aides! Green vegetable such as spinach are good to add as well to aide in healing.

The next thing you should eliminate is all commercial dairy products. These are all made from homogenized milk which is heated to 160 degrees to kill off all of the potential bad bacteria in the milk. Unfortunately, the good bacteria is killed also which renders a lot of these products very hard to digest. Lacto-intolerance is a symptom of this devitalized milk.

Raw cow's milk on the other hand is actually extremely healing and good for you! By raw I mean straight from the cow to you. This type of milk is loaded with friendly bacteria and enzymes and has less of a chance of getting spoiled by bad bacteria because of the billions of good bacteria in it. You can make it even more healing by making homemade yogurt and kefir from it.

Also, avoid anything fermented in white vinegar as it is too acidic.

<u>**THE ESSENTIAL DIET**</u>

This section is called the "Essential Diet" as these foods should be the foundation of what you eat. It took us two years of this type of diet to get to a full state of healing as my sons Crohn's was fairly advanced and with a teenager, was not easy. We were not perfect but still stayed consistent with as many of these essentials on a daily basis as possible.

The trick in beating Crohn's is to eat LOTS of food rich in friendly bacteria and live enzymes. These are the key to healing the colon and small intestines along with herbs which I will cover in the next chapter. We are trying to heal the intestines by introducing lots of friendly bacteria and enzymes and re-building the intestinal walls with pure nutrients and mineral rich foods.

Enzymatic live foods include: kefir, live yogurt, kombucha tea, sour cream, sauerkraut, miso soup, kimchee (or any fermented vegetables including pickles), raw apple cider vinegar, feta cheese, tempeh and sourdough bread. Raw unpasteurized milk was suggested but we decided not to do it as my son tested high for allergies to milk and did not want to create more uncomfortable symptoms for him.

Rebuilding foods should be rich in vitamins and minerals. These include: Bone Broth (recipe in back), raw vegetable juices, alfalfa sprouts (other sprouts may be too rough depending on what stage of healing you are in), raw apple cider vinegar, miso soup and baked chicken or rare steak if you eat meat. Feta cheese is also very rich in enzymes and can be tolerated if there is no severe allergy to milk.

Medicinal foods that fight the harmful bacteria and help with symptoms include: raw ginger, onions and garlic (can be added to your vegetable juice or bone broth soup), cold pressed extra-virgin olive oil, turmeric (anti-inflammatory) and raw apple cider vinegar.

Note that I have listed raw apple cider vinegar three times as it is essential to this diet and has tremendous health benefits! It is rich in minerals, enzymes, friendly bacteria and kills yeast, bad bacteria and parasites.

It has to be RAW. That means uncooked, live vinegar with stuff floating around on the bottom of it. The only raw apple cider vinegar I use is Braggs as it is the only one I know of that is indeed raw. All other off the shelf kind should be avoided unless you know for sure it has not been cooked!

The bottom line is start light and build into other foods over time as you heal and can handle more. It is essential to keep the colon clean and clear so eating light food with lots of enzymes is best. It will not only break down and eliminate old fecal matter but also heal the tissue that has been damaged by the disease and re-populate friendly bacteria.

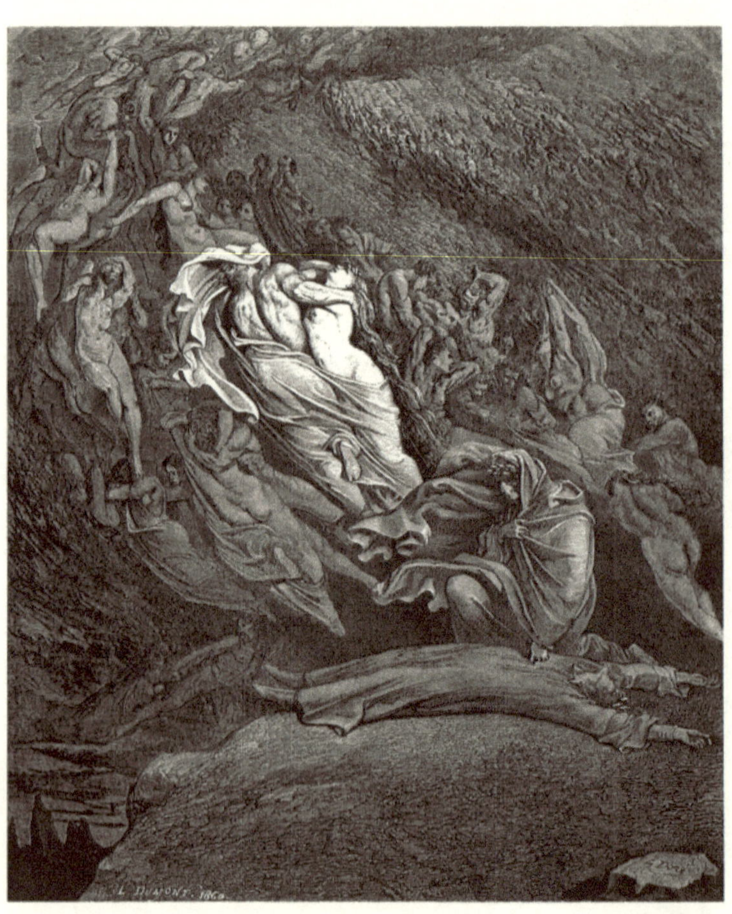

HERBS & SUPPLEMENTS

Herbs and supplements are a key component to beating this disease. While diet provides the basic nutrients and enzymes necessary to rebuild tissue and restore friendly bacteria into the intestines, herbs and supplements provide a strong synthesis of potency for targeting specific areas for healing in the body and add components that the body cannot derive from any other source.

It is essential to stick to the daily dosages for at least two weeks to see any results from using herbal medicine. If you forget to take a dose, don't get discouraged! Keep going and stick with it. It is best to do a regimen for 2 to 4 weeks and then take a break for a few weeks thereafter. This allows the body to register the healing that has taken place and allows you to see if you need to continue using it. If the symptoms return, go back on the specific herb for that area. If not, discontinue use of that particular herb.

Start by following the dosage on the bottle. Try the standard dosage for about a week and if you do not feel a difference, up it. For example, if the standard dose is to take two in the morning and you don't feel any difference, try taking two in the evening as well. You can even take two, three times a day with meals depending on the severity of your symptoms and the particular herb/supplement. I will list the dosages we used but keep in mind this was for a 14 year old boy that weighed around 100 pounds so you may need to adjust the dosages accordingly.

Note: this should only be done with the herbs listed in this book. Please research any other herbs before doing this as some high dosages of herbs such as Goldenseal, can damage the liver!

Pay attention to the milligrams and know that oils and tinctures are way more synthesized than the raw herb or tea and should be used with caution. It's all about balance. Herbs work slowly over time, so do not be in a rush to see changes. Just be consistent and make it part of your daily routine.

Also, if you venture outside of the recommendations in this book, research the herb thoroughly before using it for your healing process as some herbs contradict one another.   I also recommend researching herbs and supplements in this book if you decide to venture outside the

suggested dosage to make sure it is safe.   Some herbs and/or
supplements may contradict other things you may be taking such as
pharmaceutical or over the counter drugs if you are in the transition
process. Use the herbs and supplements moderately if this is the case.

*The following regimen was followed by a 14 year old weighing app. 100
pounds.*

ESSENTIAL ENZYMATIC FOODS

- Raw Cow's Milk
- Kefir
- Yogurt - Make sure it is the live kind
- Feta Cheese
- Sauerkraut
- Raw Apple Cider Vinegar - Use as a salad dressing or in a drink
- Sour Dough Bread
- Papaya - Fresh or dried
- Sour Pickles
- Kombucha
- Miso
- Kimchee
- Tempeh
- Sour Cream

ESSENTIAL OTHER FOODS

- Bone Broth
- Organic Meat
- Organic Fruit
- Organic Vegetables
- Raw Garlic - *Natural antibiotic and anti-parasitic*
- Raw Onions - *Natural anti-biotic and anti-parasitic*
- Extra Virgin Cold Pressed Olive Oil
- Raw Vegetable Juices – such as carrot/spinach/beet

<u>SUPPLEMENTS</u>

- Blue-Green Algae
- Bromelin - *Natural anti-inflammatory*
- Quercetin - *Natural anti-inflammatory*
- Peppermint – for pain
- Turmeric - Natural anti-inflammatory
- Ginger - Digestive Aide
- Grapefruit Seed Extract - Natural Antibiotic
- Oil of Oregano - Natural antibiotic

<u>OTHER ANTI-INFLAMMATORIES</u>

QBC Complex

- Quercetin
- Bromelin
- Vitamin C

Health food stores carry many brands of this. Take the combination 2 in the morning, 2 at night. Add an additional 2 at lunch for severe symptoms.

Turmeric

Add to food or put the powdered herb in gel caps. Take 1 to 2 at each meal.

GI Encaps

- Marshmallow
- Plantain
- Licorice Root
- Slippery Elm

This combination is sold in Health Food stores. 2 in the morning, 2 at night.

<u>**ANTI-PARASITICS**</u>

Senna

2 at night once a week for 4 weeks, off for 4 weeks, back on for 4 weeks.
Do this 2 to 3 times a year.

Wormwood

1 Dropper full of tincture with the Senna once a week with same regimen as above.

<u>**ANTI-BACTERIALS**</u>

Grapefruit Seed Extract

Oil of Oregano

Alternate GSE 3 caps 3 X Day for 2 weeks and switch to OOO 3 caps 3 X Day for 2 weeks for a total of 1 month. Rest 1 month.
Do cycle again if symptoms persist.

Can be upped to 4 /4 X Day or 5/5x day in severe cases.

This should only be done alternating 1 week of GSE and one week of OOO then breaking for one week.

** Long term use of Oil of Oregano can be damaging to the liver and wipe out friendly bacteria so during the breaks up your probiotic foods and supplements and make sure you take breaks from it in between sessions*

<u>**RESTORE & HEAL**</u>

- **Glutamine -** 2 in the morning 2 at night

- **Colostrum -** 2 in the morning 2 at night

- **Fish Oil -** 2 in the morning 2 at night

- **Cod Liver Oil -** 2 in the morning 2 at night

- **Aloe Vera Juice -** Drink daily as much as you want – minimum 1 cup

- **Digestive Enzymes** – 2 with every meal

- **Raw Apple Cider Vinegar** – 1 tbsp 3 x Day ½ hour before meals. Mix with 1 cup cold water and dilute for easier drinking

- **Acidophilus -** 3 caps 3 X Day or 1 tsp of liquid 3 x Day

<u>**PAIN RELIEF**</u>

- **Peppermint Oil** - 2 capsules with onset of pain. No more than 6 evenly spread throughout the day.

- **Ginger Root** - Boil root and drink as tea mixed with honey & lemon or add raw to juice

- **Catnip Tea** - Drink tea/herb liberally. Only buy organic catnip made for humans from the herb or health food store.

- **Magnesium Citrate** - Mix 1 tablespoon of powder into cold water and drink 1 to 3 times a day. This one really cleans your colon out so gauge your doses by what you need to do that day!

THE THERAPIES

Therapy is an expression for anything that heals body, mind and soul. When suffering from Crohn's, you need to do all three. The following therapies are listed in order of importance.

COLONICS

Colon hydrotherapy has been used for centuries for health benefits. It is essentially like taking a shower on the inside of your body. The therapy is performed by a colonics therapist on a special table where warm water is used to clean out the colon using a rectal tube. It is far more powerful than an enema as the water is continually flowing and breaking up old fecal matter, parasites, fermentation, gas and harmful bacteria that may be present in the colon. Many traditional doctors will argue that it is impossible for the colon to get impacted but this is not true. I have fasted and done colonics and enemas for many years and I am always shocked at what comes out. It is unbelievable how much better I feel after as well!

The colon can store wrong food choices from as early as infancy. White flour especially can line the colon like plaster and build up over many years as can dairy. Combine this with tons of sugar that feeds parasites we pick up from not washing our fruits and vegetables, flies landing on our food, going barefoot in yucky mud or meat that has sat out too long. Ironically, parasites reside mostly on organic produce as there is no pesticide to kill them! It is of utmost importance to wash all vegetables and fruits before eating, even if they have a peel. Also washing our hands before every meal is important as we can pick up all kinds of things just by going into public places like the gym.

Parasites are actually one of the leading causes of common ailments such as head and muscle aches, poor vision, nausea and weakness. Again, I know this from what I have experienced with my own body. I plan on writing a book just on colon cleansing because boy do I have some stories about parasites! But I can tell you that most people suffer from these entities as they can go undetected for a persons whole life if efforts are not made to eliminate them.

To get the most benefit out of your colonic, it is good to take a colon cleanser the night before such as senna. Magnesium is also good and is gentler if regular cleansers are too painful.

It is important that you learn how to hold the water inside of your colon until it fills up with as much water as possible. The longer and more water you hold inside, the more you will eliminate.

It is recommended to do a colonic series of 10 going at least once a week and supplementing with enemas in between. Take acidophilus always directly after to restore the friendly bacteria and keep eating your probiotic foods liberally. By practicing this therapy, the healing of your intestines will happen much more rapidly and effectively.

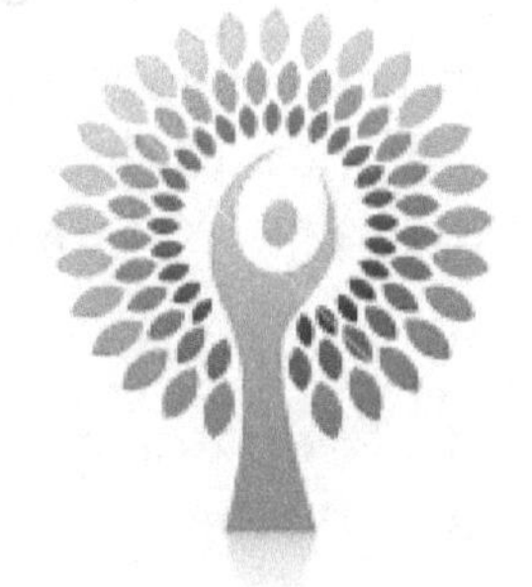

<u>**ENEMAS**</u>

Enemas are in my opinion one of the best ways to cleanse your body. It is the best and most direct way to inject your system with essential detoxing aides and friendly bacteria depending on what you use. I know that sounds crazy but the benefits you reap when you do it are phenomenal! I have a small bucket with a tube that my colonics therapist gave me years ago and I love to experiment with different concoctions for different ailments. What is fascinating is that the colon is networked into every organ of the body so you can target different areas by what you use in your water.

Most local pharmacy's carry enema bags. The most basic form of doing an enema is using warm water. Cold water will cause cramping so avoid that if possible. Lie on your left side and allow the water to fill that side up. As you feel it filling, roll over on your back and then onto your right side, all the while letting the water flow. If you feel an urge to go, stop and allow your body to eliminate what it will. The more water you hold inside the better but it takes practice and it also depends on what sort of detoxification your body is going through.

I recommend doing enemas every night before bed followed by a hot sea salt or bentonite clay bath but if this is not possible, at least once a week.   The salt or clay bath continue to draw out the toxins and is a nice treat after, especially if you have some cramping.

Cramping is normal but you have to gauge yourself and only do what you can. It is recommended to keep going with the water until it comes out clean but sometimes it is too much.

I try to do at least 4 buckets per session but have done as many as 8. At least do one to start but know the more you do, the better the results! Also, drink tons of water during the process to help the body filter out the toxins and flush them through. Hot catnip or peppermint tea is also good to drink during the process to relieve cramping.

Once you get that down, try adding some ingredients to your water. I have many recipes for this but I will focus on what is good for Crohn's specifically for now.

Aloe Vera Juice

Add a cup of Aloe Vera Juice to your water for each round for extra emulsion and healing power.

Raw Apple Cider Vinegar

Add a tablespoon or two to each round of your session to kill yeast, and bacteria and add friendly bacteria back into your intestines. This miracle juice also alkalinizes the body making it less acidic and less friendly for parasites to live in.

Catnip Tea

Use the tea straight by making a big batch on the stove. Make sure it cools way down first to a warm tea by using ice, Aloe or just letting it sit a few hours to cool down. Great for headaches, muscle tension, candida and stomach pain. Try drinking some of it too while you do your session for maximum results.

Coffee

Bring a large pot of water to a boil and add organic coffee grounds to it as if you were making it to drink. Allow to cool to a warm temperature. If you plan on adding ice to cool it down, make it stronger than usual. Use straight as an enema going at least four rounds. Great for detoxing the liver. My eyesight even got better on this one!

<u>**COUNSELING**</u>

Having Crohn's can make you feel depressed, alone and separate from your friends and family because it is such a unique experience that only someone who is living with it really understands. It can interfere with everyday activities that your average person takes for granted.

I fully believe that body, mind and spirit are all connected and you should treat and heal all three to get fully well. I highly recommend getting some kind of counseling from a professional whom you can outpour your frustration to and work through the challenges that you are facing with this disease.

Often we try and do this with the ones we love but I've found that it is healthier to have someone whom is neutral and unemotionally involved to be your listening board.

Not to say you shouldn't share with your family and friends but use the therapy more for the core issues that may be present.

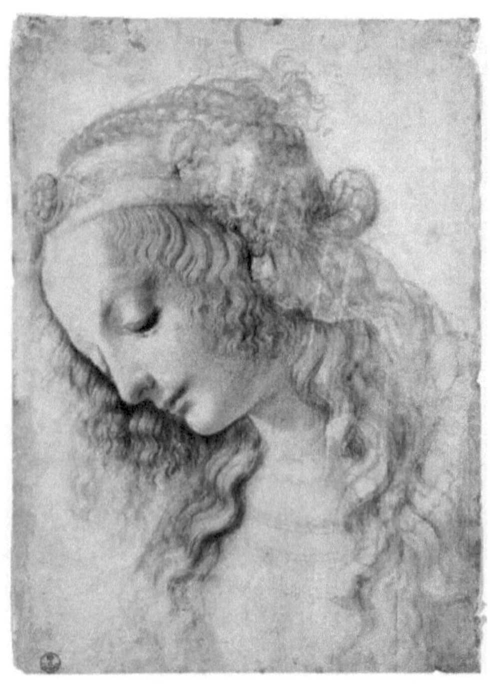

<u>**THE RECIPES**</u>

<u>**APPLE CIDER VINEGAR DRINK**</u>

Add one tablespoon of Raw Apple Cider Vinegar to an 8 ounce glass of water. Drink first thing in the morning and/or after every meal.

<u>**BONE BROTH**</u>

1 whole free-range chicken
4 quarts cold filtered water
2 tablespoons raw apple cider vinegar
1 large onion, coarsely chopped
2 carrots, peeled and coarsely chopped
3 celery stalks, coarsely chopped
1 bunch parsley

Note: Farm-raised, free-range chickens give the best results. Non free range raised chickens will not produce stock that gels.

Cut chicken parts into several pieces including the neck and wings cut into several pieces. Place chicken in a large stainless steel pot with water, vinegar and all vegetables except parsley.

Let stand 30 minutes to 1 hour. Bring to a boil, and remove scum that rises to the top. Reduce heat, cover and simmer for 6 to 8 hours. The longer you cook the stock, the richer and more flavorful it will be. About 10 minutes before finishing the stock, add parsley. This will infuse additional minerals to the broth.

Remove whole chicken or pieces with a slotted spoon. If you are using a whole chicken, let cool and remove chicken meat from the carcass. Reserve for other uses, such as chicken salads, enchiladas, sandwiches or curries.

Strain the stock into a large bowl and reserve in your refrigerator until the fat rises to the top and congeals. Skim off this fat and reserve the stock in covered containers in your refrigerator or freezer.

Drink with meals or use to cook with. Very mineral rich and healing to the stomach. Beef and fish bones can be used as well with same recipe above.

HOMEMADE SAUERKRAUT

1 Medium Head of Cabbage
1-3 Tbsp. <u>sea salt</u>

- **Chop** or **shred** cabbage. **Sprinkle** with salt.

- Add 1 tsp of caraway seeds to add flavor (optional)

- **Knead** the cabbage with clean hands, or **pound** with a potato masher or Cabbage Crusher about 10 minutes, until there is enough liquid to cover.

- **Stuff** the cabbage into a quart jar, **pressing** the cabbage underneath the liquid. If necessary, add a bit of water to completely cover cabbage.

- **Cover** the jar with a tight lid, airlock lid, or coffee filter secured with a rubber band.

- **Culture** at room temperature (60-70°F is preferred) for **at least 2 weeks** until desired flavor and texture are achieved. If using a tight lid, **burp daily** to release excess pressure.

- Once the sauerkraut is finished, **put a tight lid on the jar** and **move to cold storage**. The sauerkraut's flavor will continue to develop as it ages.

RAW COW MILK YOGURT

1 quart fresh raw milk
2 tbsp Bulgarian or Greek starter OR
2 tbsp yogurt from a previous batch OR
2 tbsp plain, unsweetened, ORGANIC yogurt with live active cultures

- Heat milk in a saucepan ON medium until it reaches about 110° F

- Remove from heat and whisk in 2 tablespoons starter culture or use two tablespoons yogurt to inoculate the raw milk.

- Using either a yogurt maker, dehydrator or slow cooker set the temperature to 110° Fahrenheit / 43° Celsius and allow it to culture for eight to twelve hours.

- Once the culturing period of eight to twelve hours is complete, place it in the refrigerator to chill and solidify for at least one hour

- Sweeten if desired, with honey or maple syrup or add vanilla extract or fruit puree for flavor.

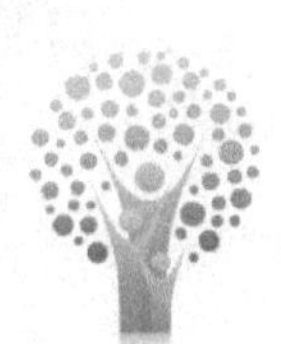

<u>**CONCLUSION**</u>

I hope that you have found this book to be informative and helpful. This is the regimen we followed for 2 solid years and ended up symptom free for nearly 10 years now!

Only you know for sure what is right for your body as long as you listen! I know it is along rough road but there is light at the end of the tunnel and with persistence and hopeful vision; you can heal your body!

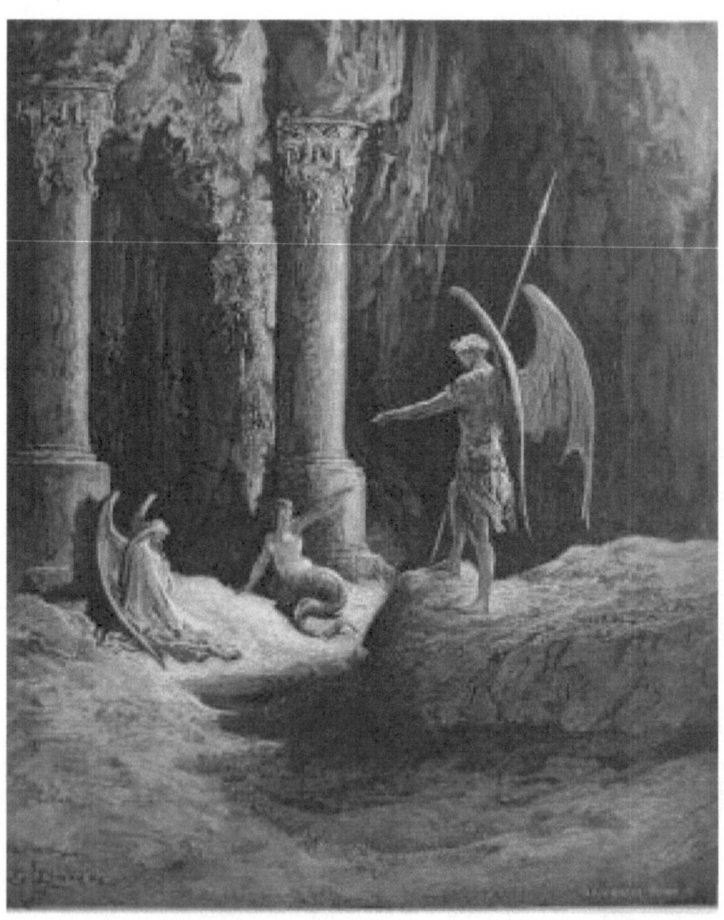

www.ingramcontent.com/pod-product-compliance
Lightning Source LLC
Chambersburg PA
CBHW051406250726
48656CB00006B/2291